BEING FIT

MANAV BHATT

ISBN 978-1-63997-049-0

"TO MY PARENTS AND ALL THOSE

WHO INSPIRED ME."

Contents

Contents

PREFACE

My book is based on the important key points of fitness. Its my personel belief that our body is the only thing in which we have to live in, so its our duty to keep it healthy, I have tried to cover all small and important points related to fitness, which most of the people needs to know and I have converted my experience and some knowledge here in short and simple words by not making it complicated to make it easy for the readers to read it in one go, Besides fitness, there has always been a perception of mine about success, which I think of to let it flow by writing it in the stream of Words.

Acknowledgements

This book is the first masterpiece of mine, its been a fantastic journey in writing this books and there had been a alot of research being done by me. So, first of all I would like to thank my parents for believing in me, A big thanks to all of my readers for giving your precious time to read my book or just taking a glimpse of my book. And I would like to thank the Notionpress.com for publishing my book and giving this wonderful platform to the people like me who needed a direction to write

Content

I

What made me to start excersing?

Back in the days when I was in 7th std, we used to have the history of Indian warriors with their pictures in our book, and history has always been my favourite subject. So I started to gain more knowledge about this warriors from the internet.

After knowing them completely I also got to know that the physique of this warriors were used to be very strong and they used to have their height saddles of 6-7 feets, and I was very curious to know the secrets of their power. As an innocent child I asked my father to solve this query of mine, as how and what made them so strong and my father explained to me about the exercise and fitness routines they used to follow in the olden times for conditioning of their body. And he also told me that it was very important for them to keep their body strong because, they used to fight against the enemy in the warfield with their heavy armours and its not a piece of cake for everyone to lift that heavy armours. Listening to him I got to know the importance of fitness and I got inspired and felt motivated and I also decided to make myself in proper shape by starting exercises. For this I started searching on youTube to get knowledge of different exercises and their impacts, and I started to do some normal exercises like pushups, squats, crunches by following youtube videos and fitness motivational videos, as a beginner it was difficult for me to do this exercises because after one day I was exhausted like hell and my legs were literally screaming due to pain, my mind was saying not to continue on the next day but my father made me understand that the "the pain today is a relief in your future". Next day I continued to do exercise, after some days of regular work out I started observaing changes in myself in terms of performance, muscle growth, I gradually started feeling energetic and increasing my strength, frequency and endurance, and that made me swell full of positiveness and then I never stopped and tried to keep myself persistence in fitness till today after 4 years. Fitness has changed me alot in terms of my attitude, my focus, and many health benefits. Exercise is a type of wall between me and stress. I am very thankful to God for giving intuition within me by which I could start building up my fitness.

II

What is fitness?

By hearing the word "fitness" som e of us might get thoughts of a body which is full shredded and muscular and we imagine about that hard work and all that stuff, that's because of characters and imaginations that we have made about fitness by watching movies of our favourite heroes with muscular body like Tiger shroff, Hrithik roshan etc. But thats not a quoted physique by which we can say that he is very fit because he has six pack abs and long head biceps. Its not mandatory to have six pack abs to call yourself as fit person, its all about the perception, stamina, the food you eat, and exercises you do.

My wish is to see every Indian to be fit and to spread importance of fitness and making its concept very clear. Because, In these advanced world, machines have made humans lazy to an extent that they think twice even about getting up and taking up the glass of water for themselves. I am not criticising the technologies, Yes they have made our work easy by fulfilling the communication gap and many other problems that used to have in the olden times, instead I am just trying to say that, getting addicted to the automatic machines can also cause harm. Because it cuts off our maximum physical work. I laughed imagining that in today's times a person daily drives his/her car to a gym to just walk on a tredmill, instead he/she can go by walking and half of the warm up will get done while reaching there.

The one who understands the concept of fitness properly, could make the life very healthy and can swell full of positiveness. Physical fitness is generally achieved through moderate or vigorous exercises, proper nutritions and proper rest. Any exercise program should include cardiovascular **exercise**, which strengthens the heart and burns calories. It is not compulsory to join gym if you want a athletic physique, you can also achieve it by doing effective exercises at your home or garden or wherever you feel comfortable but doing exercises in open air can enhance your mood and boosts your performance. Meaning of exercise is not only resistance trainings like pushups, lifting dumbells, crunches etc. A simple jog or walk for 1 hour or cycling for 1 hour can also helps you to maintain your physique.

III

Sedantary lifestyle

A sedentary lifestyle is a lifestyle in which there is a little or no physical activity involved in simple words we can say that a person who is very lazy is living in its sedentary lifestyle, this type of persons are sitting or lying all the time and engaged in the activity like using social media, playing games, Watching movies etc. The person living in sedentary lifestyle have higher chances of illness and problems like increasing weight, joints pain etc. Sedentary behavior is not the same as physical inactivity: sedentary behavior is defined as "any waking behavior characterized by an energy expenditure less than or equal to 1.5 metabolic equivalents (METs), while in a sitting, reclining or lying posture". This can even cause death sometimes. At least 300,000 premature deaths, and $90 billion in direct healthcare costs are caused by obesity and sedentary lifestyle per year in the US alone, so we can think how much would be the death rate world wide, this is all because of lack of fitness. The main thing which maximum people faces is laziness before starting exercise that is why they couldn't stay consistent in it, but we have to understand that before giving pressure to our body by exercising we have to tackle our laziness and think about our fitness goal and working on it to get better results. Yes, there is hard work but remember one thing "no pain, no gain" thats your attitude which makes the difference. Every successful person or every athletes or bodybuilders have sweated for their success.

IV
Yoga

This is very common word "yoga" which you have heard many a times, and which you have seen how Swami Ramdev perfoming on T.V channels. But do you really know the importance of it? Yoga was originated in ancient India by our ancestors which simple means the group exercise of our lungs, mental and spiritual health. Yoga is one f the six orthodox philosophical schools of Hinduism. There are a broad variety of yoga schools, practices, and goals in Hinduism, Buddhism, and Jainism and there are four paths or types of yoga: Karm yoga, Kriya yoga, Bhakti yoga, and Jnana yoga. Research studies have shown that traditional yoga systems that include breathing exercises and asanas or postures, chants, and meditation can reduce stress and improve immunity and lung functions. Traditional forms and modern methods of yoga are practiced worldwide. The first Hindu teacher to actively advocate and disseminate aspects of yoga, not including asanas, to a western audience, Swami Vivekananda, toured Europe and the United States in the 1890s.

There are many benefits of yoga but here are the top most:

1. Increase your flexibility
2. Increase your immune system
3. Yoga helps to keep your joints active.
4. Its a powerful mindfulness practice.
5. Increase oxygen level in blood.

My personal experience of yoga was very beneficial,when I was suffering from acute bronchitis, I started practicing yoga on daily basis and it has helped me alot to cure my pain. So its very important for us to keep our body fit from within also.

V
Meditation

Practice of meditation have been carried out in Indian culture since ancient times which was used to perform by rishi munis to focus on the devotion of god basically it is a type of practice where we sit and close our eyes and try to focus on breathing, or any other object, thought or activity. Its very important topic to discuss on, because this habit has to implemented by everyone in there life, it helps our mind to focus on our goal by not getting distracted and it is very useful for the ones who can't concentrate on their studies or any work. Many neurological studies have found that meditation helps to alleviate mental and physical conditions, such as reducing depression, stress and anxiety.

There are many emotional benefits of meditaion:

1. You can build skill to manage any stress.

2. You will start focusing on present.

3. Creativity skill.

4. You will start noticing changes in your patience level, and your perception for life will get change.

5. Negative emotions will reduce.

VI

Early to rise

There is an old saying, "early to bed and early to rise", but are we actually following that? When it comes to exercise, everyone has their different schedules and their work out times may varied like some of us may do at evening while some of us may do at afternoon but the best time do any form of exercise is after waking up early in the morning, reason is that because exercising on an empty stomach could burn more fat and you will get results more quicker, other thing is that if you exercise in the early morning, it means you're less prone to distractions. When you first wake up you have haven't started tackilng your day to day's list, you are also less likely to get phone call, messages, and emails. So you can completely focus on your exercise without any disturbance. You can go for jogging or cycling after waking up, and can make yourself being exposed to morning sunrays to get vitamin-D. You will feel the positiveness of exercising for all day long, and can do some other work at the time of your previous work out schedule.

VII

Fitness in olden times

There were no gyms or any advanced equipments for exercises during olden times or during medieval times, Akhara or Akhada is a Indian word for a place of soil(mitti) where people were used to train their physique by doing vyayama(exercises), kusthi, malakhamba, sword training etc their daily training were so hard that's the main reason why the warriors of India were so strong by their physique because they used to carry heavy swords and wear heavy armours of 45-50 kg on their chest and they used to fight in war all day long by wearing all this heavy stuff, so their body got used to it, we have seen the pictures of Indian warriors like Maharana Pratap, Chhatrapti Shivaji Maharaj also warriors in Mahabharata like karna, Arjuna and many others, endowed with resplendent bodies, whose feats of strength, endurance, and their diet were very rich in protien and other required nutritions.

VIII

Kalaripayattu(Indian martial art)

As martial art is a form of fitness, do you know our Indian martial art? which is known as Kalaripayattu, most of the people have heard it for the first time. Kalaripayattu also known simply as kalari, which is originated from modern day Kerala, which lies on the southwest coast of India. It is believed to be the oldest surviving martial art with a history of spanning more than 3000 years. Kalaripayattu is mentioned in the Vadakkan Pattukal, a collection of ballads written about the Chekavar of the Malabar region of Kerala. Kalaripayattu is a martial art designed for the ancient battlefield (the word "Kalari" meaning "battlefield"), with weapons and combative techniques that are unique to India. According to some legends, Parashurama is believed to have learned this art from Lord Shiva, and Parashurama is believed to have taught this art to the original settlers of Kerala, and credits him with the establishment of the first 108 kalaris in Kerala, along with the instruction of the first 21 Kalaripayattu gurus in Kerala on the destruction of enemies. It is condisered one of the best way of keeping the body fit and stretchable because there are so many different moves and skills in this wonderful art. In today's times all are promoting kung fu and karate but no one is promoting our Indian arts like Kalaripayattu, kusthi, malakhamba, these are our prides and we should respect this ancient arts and we should spread this art in the world by spreading the knowledge of it.

IX

Nutritions and diet

Proper physical fitness is not just by doing exercises because it is incomplete without proper nutritions and a sensible diet, its a fuel for your fitness. You can have a healthy body weight and good body fat percentage through proper diet. A clean, vegan and healthy diet will offer a better you. You will find yourself changing in terms of stamina and endurance once you start planning your diet. There are **seven**main classes of **nutrients**that the body needs. These are carbohydrates, proteins, fats, vitamins, minerals, fibre and water. It is important that everyone consumes these **seven nutrients**on a daily basis to help them build their bodies and maintain their health. In these, protien and carbohydrates are very important nutrients for our body, protien helps our muscles to repair all the tissues and allow muscles to grow and carbohydrates helps our body to grow. **Fats in food**come in several forms, including saturated, monounsaturated, and polyunsaturated. Too much **fat**or too much of the wrong type of **fat**can be unhealthy. Some examples of **foods**that contain **fats**are butter, oil, nuts, meat, fish, and some dairy products, but as much as possible it is good to stay away from bad fats like butter and oil instead we can eat ghee with milk because it makes our bones and joints strong.

X

Sports

Sports are the best are st way to keep yourself active, it can be any explosive sports which demands more stamina, reflexes, endurance such as football, badminton, cricket etc. Playing outdoor games and running helps our body to sleep well, allows digestion process to carry out its function smoothly, develops our cardiovascular muscles and makes our heart healthy. The more active a person is, the more calories the person will burn. Fitness helps in preventing fat to be accumulated in the body and reducing the risk of obesity and obesity-related diseases. Sports also helps you to practice the co-ordination of your mind with your hands and legs. If you are sporty then you are more likely to have a healthy lifestyle.

XI

Eating kachra, junk food

Yes, junk food is one of the biggest enemy of your fitness goal, exercising hard and not following the proper diet by eating junk food will give you nothing, instead it will looks like that you are working hard to just eat that junk food which is full of sugar, salts and carbohydrates and your hardwork simply goes worthless. When junk food is consumed very often, the excess fat, simple carbohydrates, and processed sugar found in junk food contributes to an increased risk of obesity, cardiovascular disease, and many other chronic health conditions.

I know it makes our mind to get distracted towards it but once we understand that eating that junk food is no where beneficial to us than we can just grab our fitness goals easily.

XII

What Ayurveda says about fitness?

Ancient Ayurvedic scripts written by our ancestors have mentioned that moving body is very important and it is essential to do physical exercises on the daily basis.

Ayurveda has only mentioned about the necessity of doing exercises, it has not been mentioned that which type of exercise we should to do, in short you can do whatever exercise you enjoy. In the sequence of the daily routine, exercise comes after anointing one's body with oil. One place where we see this practice is a traditional Indian martial arts form called Kalaripayattu, which is practiced in Kerala. The reasoning behind this is that when you anoint your body with oil, there's more flexibility, which results in fewer injuries. Here was the perception of ayurvedic script towards fitness now lets talk about the importance of Indian ayurveda. Basically, ayurveda is the traditional hindu systems of medicines of herbal treatment. In Sanskrit ayurveda means "the science of life", because it helps to cure a particular disease in a traditional way by using natural medicines like turmeric, ginger, tulsi, aloe vera and many more. Ayurvedic knowledge originated in India more than 5000 years ago, it is often called as the "mother of all healing" previously the knowledge of ayurveda were used to give by the accomplished masters to their disciples, in this way ayurvedic knowledge passed from one generation to another. But it is not valued by most of the people by not giving importance to the heritage of Indian ayurveda inspite we are using allopathy medicines instead of ayurvedic medicines for the sake of quick relief.

XIII
Neurological benefits of exercise.

Whenever you perform any exercise or form of exercises like running, cycling, swimming, playing any sport your heart beat increases and your heart starts pumping more blood and oxygen to the brain and it aids to release hormones which helps to make more brain cells and it also supports plasticity to your brain to make more cell connections in its cortical areas. It also produce hormones which reduces body stress level like adrenaline and cortisol, it also stimulates the production of endorphins which is body's natural painkiller and mood enhancer. Endorphins also trigger a positive feeling in the body

XIV

Rest

Rest is very important from the point of view of muscle growth because your muscles needs rest too. when you start working out your body break downs glycogen to make fuel for your workout and your muscle tissues starts breaking through tiny cracks and this cracks heals when you are sleeping because your body stays in complete rest at night, this process of muscle breaking and healing is called as hypertrophy. Hypertrophy allows your muscles to grow slowly, in other words hypertrophy is response to exercise. This process makes your muscle bigger and allows to accumulate more structural contractile protiens.

XV

Hydration

Its important to replace fluids which is lost through sweating process during workout and the best fluid is water. When you are dehydrated your body and mind cannot function properly, and your body will show symptoms of dehydration like dark urine and lack of sweat when exercising. Staying hydrated is very important because the food you eat get converted into glycogen to heal our muscle tissues and this process needs water to run it smoothly.

If you don't drink enough fluid:

1. Your body temperature and heart rate will get increase, if your hydration level is below the required level.

2. Your enery level will fall down and you will feel tired.

3. You may feel stomach discomfort because of gastric emptying.

4. It decreased skin elasticity.

5. Low blood pressure.

XVI

Detoxification of body.

Detoxification is the process in which toxic substances are eliminated form our body, generally this process is mainly carried out by liver. Fortunately, your body is well-equipped to eliminate toxins and doesn't require special diets or expensive supplements to do so. While diet for detoxing will do nothing that your body will do automatically if you follow this points.

1. Reduce alocohol

90% of alcohol is metabolised in live and excessive consumption can damage your liver resulting in disfunction of the liver by not filtering waste and other toxins in the body. This will lead to inflammation of liver which will increase toxins level in your body.

2. Sleep well

Focusing on your sleep can help your body to detoxify toxins properly, because when your body is in rest your brain reorganised and recharge itself, as well as remove toxic byproduct that have collected throughout the day.

3. Stay hydrated

Water regulates your body temperature, lubricates joints, aids digestion and nutrients absorption and detoxify your body by waste products.

4. Stop eating sugar and processed foods.

Sugar and processed food which is easily available in shops are said to be the root of all public health issue. It is been linked with to obesity and chronic disease like heart disease, diabetes and cancer. These disease slowly stops the natural ability of your body to detoxify the toxic materials.

XVII
High Intensity Interval Trainig(HIIT)

It is a form of cardiovascular exercise strategy which is usually done in short period of recovery time, until you are too exhausted to continue. **HIIT workouts**provide improved athletic capacity and condition as well as improved glucose metabolism.

Benefits of interval training:

1. It quickly burns your calories and can help you to become shredded or in weight loss.

2. It increases metabolism and elevate your body endurance.

3. It improves heart health

4. It may also help to improve the measures of blood pressure, blood sugar levels, and cholesterol. The reason I have mentioned this exercise is because I have been doing this exercise to maintain my physique and I personally find

it very effective, but remember excessive makes it worst because it can also damage your heart artery if done vigorously, so my advice is to do it 2 or 3 times a week to get results.

XVIII

Why men skip legs day?

We shouldn't forgot that half of the body is our leg, so it is equally important to train them as our upper body. Most of the men skip leg days because of the pain, generally it is hard to train our legs because it demands a lot pain that you can't even walk on your legs after the workout. But muscular leg or strong leg will give you a maintained and attractive physique. It can also increase your overall balance. For those who participate in sports, strengthening your **legs**will help with many skills such as jumping, running, and other **powerful**movements that are of vital **importance**to your performance. Weak legs will slow down your performance because legs are dominatly used in all exercises. Strong legs will help you in deadlifts and prevent injuries in spine. If you are playing any sports like cricket or football your speed will surely get increased.

XIX

Effects of testosterone on your perfomance.

Testosteroneis the primary sex hormone and anabolic steroid in males. It increases the levels of growth hormones in response to exercise, it also increases the red blood cell count produced in the bone marrow. If you have a low level of fitness you are likely to have a greater increase in testosterone response to exercise. As your body adjusts to the demands of exercise the testosterone response will decrease.

Natural ways to boost your testosterone:

Although there are supplements available in shops to boosts your testosterone level but my recommendation is to boost it by natural way.

1. Lifting weights makes your body to release more testosterone.

2. Expose yourself more to sunlight.

3. Eat protien, good fat and carbohydrates.
4. Say no to masturbation.
5. Take plenty of rest.

XX
Things to avoid

Proper health and fitness relfect a mature decision you make. There are some habits which should be avoided by you if you want to see yourself fit for long period of time.

Alcohol:

Many people in our society have accepted the fact that drinking alcohol gives you self confidence, and it is stress relief, but it reality this people are digging their own grave by consuming alcohol. Alcohol can slow down your metabolism and weaken your muscles and give you fatigue. Excessive consumption of alcohol can not only affects your fitness goal, infact it ruins your whole life.

Tobacco:

Cigarettes, cigars and smokeless tobacco contain a whole gamut of cancer causing chemicals that provide no positive health effects. Our people are drawn at a wrong path because maximum people are consuming this poision. If you want your dream physique then don't make this mistake of consuming this types of poisions.

XXI
Injuries

A workout injury can occur to anyone, no matter how experienced you are or your fitness level. Injury can occur while walking also. But you can cut risks of getting injured by following some precautions,

Common workout injuries,

People hurt themselves in all kinds of ways when they workout. Common workout injuries include:

1. Ankle twist
2. Muscle pain and strain.
3. Shoulder injury.
4. Cramps.
5. Calf injuries.

Here are the precautions

Warm ups; Every single workout session should be begin with warm ups, it helps your body to get ready for the workout. Warm ups can be of any types:

1. Skipping for 5 to 10 mins.
2. Cycling.
3. Spot running.

Strecthing;

Do dynamic strecthing after warm ups it helps to get more flexibility during workout and prevent injuries.

Ease into it;

Whenever you start a new workout program, start slowly. Then gradually buil intensity, strength and frequency, because quality is more important than quantity.

XXII

Side effects of steroids

To increase muscle strength some people use substances like anabolic-androgenic steroid(AAS). This are a synthetic form of testosterone, which is the primary male sex hormone and makes muscle cells to grow and "bulk up". A variety of side effects can occur when anabolic steroids are misused, ranging from mild effects to ones that are harmful or even life-threatening. Most are reversible if the user stops taking the drugs. However, others may be permanent or semi-permanent. Most data on the long-term effects of anabolic steroids in humans come from case reports rather than formal epidemiological studies. Serious and life-threatening adverse effects may be underreported, especially since they may occur many years later. So its better to make muscles through pure nutritions & diet.

XXIII

Either kill depression or get killed by depression.

According to Bhagvad Gita "mind acts like an enemy if we don't control it" and let's talk on very important topic which is depression. This is one of the most common situation through which our most of the youngsters go through, its just because you have less trained your

mind. Just ask yourself when did you last trained your brain? If you are strong by your body and weak by your brain will be of worthless. Training of the brain in the sense means to develop self confidence, creating positive mind-set through setting your goals, self-talk, long vision, not giving up attitude. In Bhagvad Gita Lord Krishna says that the mind can be controlled through constant practice and detachment." A trained mind person will never get distracted by any other problems, instead he will just focus on his goal. I have heard many people saying this fixed line, "Man I am depressed and I am feeling very low", in reality it is just a bullshit, because a person who is working everyday to achieve his/her goal will never get depressed because there is always an excitement in their mind to grab their goals, and a person who is doing nothing all the day will get all this negative thoughts because his brain is not trained to overcome any kind of problem or situation. Your body is just a slave of your brain, it will react as per your brain will commands it and brain can be controlled by you. So instead of ruining your body by a negative mind-set, train it to help yourself to find a better you. Train your body by practicing yoga and meditation to increase your focus and exercising is the best doctor of your brain to get positiveness. Points which will train your mind and makes you happy and successful

1. Try not to give up.

2. Do more hardwork to achieve your goals.

3.Try to stay happy even when situations are not going according to you.

4. Watch or read biographies of successful peoples.

5. Label your emotions.

6. Give yourself **the**same advice you'd give to **a**trusted friend.

7. Practice gratitude.

8. Read books based on success and life.

9. Never apply shortcuts.

10. Eat well.

After all it is up to that either you want to kill depression or get killed by depression.

XXIV

How covid-19 changed the minds of people

The sudden and massive hit of Covid-19 has brought this world to a standstill, conditions of lockdown have changed the mind of people due to closure of business activities, public places, fitness and activity centers, and overall social life, has hampered many aspects of the lives of people including routine fitness activities of fitness freaks, which has resulted in various psychological issues and serious fitness and health concerns. From this maximum people have understood the importance of fitness, so they have started taking care of their health by doing exercises and by avoiding junk food. Previously people's mindset was that the body can only be maintained by going to the gym but this Covid-19 situations have changed their perception about fitness.

XXV

Will your luck decide your future?

"Let's see what has been written in my luck", this the most common line people say when they fail to do something. People often refuse to do something in which there is hardwork, why they must be doing that?

You know there are always 5 direct rules of success, no matter in whatever field you are these are applicable on every phase of your life. These are the most common rules which are followed by all successful peoples and I also have been trying to implement these in my life. Making your physique is very important but to be successful should always be your first priority. I feel that by following these rules anyone can become successful and earn respect.

1. Hardwork: Thats very simple you have to choose from these two which is, whether you want to give excuse or you want success. It is possible that you might don't have skills but if you do hardwork it is possible that you might produce your talent. There's no better way to achieve succes than hardwork.

2. Discipline: The reason why discipline is important to become successful is because if you don't have discipline then you don't deserve to be successful. Discipline is when everyday you prove your decision to be right by working on it. So rule number 2 would always be discipline.

3. Self-belief: self belief means believing on yourself. Its important to be self believed because you need to have confidence on yourself that yes I know myself and I can do anything to achieve it.

4. Obsession: There should be always be a crave for your success, You should be obsessed about your victory. When there's nothing like obsession, craziness for your goal in your mind there will no be success waiting for you.

5. Patience: This one of the most important rules for the success.For example if you have planted a seed in soil, its not only soil that will help this seed to grow there is also sunlight and water which will also help this seed to grow, and the seed will not grow in just one day. Similarly, success will not grab your feet in just one day you need to be very patient for that. This are the main rules for success which you should try to implement in your day to day life. Apart form these rules there are certain things which we also need to keep it in our mind, which I believe as very important and have worked in my life. There will always people available who will try to insult yoy and demotivates you whenever you are on the path of success, never listen to this kind of people because insult does only those who can't match your level because they feel jealous by not being you. You know there is always a different path of champions by walking on which they become legends, champions doesn't like to be a part of crowd they always make their way own their own. Always Remember this thing if you don't want to be a part of a crowd,then learn to live alone, remember

there are always people to help you out in the path of success but you have to walk alone on your own because you have chosen your field so stop taking support of others shoulder, its not your luck it is your hardwork which will decide your luck. Don't wait for bad times instead, enjoy every moment of your life, main thing is how long can you support yourself. Success doesn't see that you are rich or poor it only sees your hardwork. Legends have different ingredient in them because they have that dare to accept the challenges in life. Another thing that matters is don't blame anyone when you face any failure, take your responsibility yourself. One thing is common among all successful and legend people that they made their decision once and worked on it in their whole life that have had always made them so special. They were not born with best capabilities or best privileges but they had one speacial thing in them that is they believed in themselves and their decision. If you also have a different ingredient in you, then work on it to call yourself as legend of your field.

XXVI

Never give up

"Failures" what are the failures?, your perception about failures might be different but in reality failures are the thrust to the planet of success. Everyone among us must have faced failures a quite few times only difference is some must have faced it on bigger level and some must have faced on lower level.

That one question which every person has asked atleast once in their life is that who is responsible for your failure, I say if I have failed then I am responsible for my failure, ask yourself. If you have failed then you are responsible for it, try to first accept it. A warrior's first value is to accept their mistakes. Now you have to work so hard that your failures get converted into your success, just because you have fallen that doesn't mean that you can't get up and bounce back again, it doesn't that you can't win. So work hard to an extent that succes becomes your slave and it will only happen when you will stop blaming others and start accepting your mistakes. You don't give credits to others when you win similarly, don't blame anyone when you loose. We need to understand the main difference between a fighter and a warrior is that when a fighter or a weak person looses they blame it on his coaches or teachers, these people can never become warriors in their life because they blame others for their failures. Ask yourself if you would have won then would you have given credits to them? Whereas if warriors looses he will accept his mistakes, and he starts preparing himself by working hard. Remember, a person who is scared is the person who is not prepared. So always work so hard that success itself comes to you.

XXVII
Anger management

Anger is a matter that if you use it in a right way there is no better enery than this and if you don't use it properly it will harm you for sure. But you need to understand that you get angry, there are two things which can make you angry.

1. Weak people gets angry because they don't have the strength to handle about what people says about them.

2. The kind of people who know they can do better than this and still are not able to do it. Now you decide which kind of anger you get.Just like some people gets angry by hearing the truth when you them that they are a traitor or a buffoon, but their anger is of no use because they can't do anything about it because its a truth. Now talking about the other type/reason of getting angry, that anger was also there in Maharana pratap, Chhatrapti Shivaji Maharaj, Bhagat singh, Chandrasekhar azad and many more real heroes like this because they used their anger in a right way by converting anger into resolution and not by just smashing their head on the wall.

If you use your anger in a good way than you could convert anger into your success, the reason is why anger is important to acheive success is because sometime some must have insulted you, questioned on your integrity and it must have boosts your ego and you start working hard to become successful person to prove yourself to that particular person, history is witness take any of the examples whenever there had been an insult of any person his anger had made him to become a successful person.

Now question is that how to control our anger?

Whenever you get angry, first try keep your mind cool and ask yourself that will this anger harm anyone and will it help me to move forward and what is your loss and benefit of it. The best solution of anger is smile, yes you read it right, I am telling you the hardest thing which you can ever do when you are angry, but trust me if you will try stay quiet at that time and take a deep breathe your anger will drained out. Sometimes anger turned out to be very hazardous for our family, work or relationships, for example the nail which is hammered in the wall is very difficult to remove similarly the relationship that our ruined due to anger are very difficult to handle or get back.

Till here was my journey with you by sharing some secrets of fitness and success, this is all what I have been trying to implement in my life.

CONCLUSION

After knowing and implementing the concept of fitness and success one can achieve their bestest phase of the life, reading or watching motivational books or videos of fitness or success and not but not learning from it will be of no use. Fitness have been one of our culture since ancient times now this is our duty to carry on this culture to the generations by making them understand the importance of fitness and their benefits, and we also need to understand too. Physical activities results in increasing exercise capacity, which may lead to many heath benefits, but there has to be some discipline in it to make this far more better. By reading and following the rules mentioned above one can achieve his fitness treasure and can fulfil his fitness crave, and success path is far more harder then fitness. Fitness is a source through which our mind gets trained for the hardwork, or can say fitness is indirectly linked with success.

THANK YOU!